Stronger, Faster, Better: Mastering Your Life Through Fitness And Self Improvement

Chapter 1: Introduction
- Importance of self improvement and how the gym can be a valuable tool
- Overview of what will be covered in the book

Chapter 2: Understanding Self Improvement
- Definition of self improvement
- The benefits of self improvement
- Different areas of life to focus on for self improvement

Chapter 3: Why the Gym Matters
- The benefits of going to the gym
- How physical exercise can impact mental health and overall wellbeing
- Overview of different types of exercise and how they can benefit you

Chapter 4: Setting Goals
- The importance of setting goals for self improvement
- SMART goal setting method
- Tips for staying motivated and on track with your goals

Chapter 5: Mindset and Mindfulness
- The role of mindset in selfimprovement
- How to cultivate a growth mindset
- The benefits of mindfulness and meditation

Chapter 6: Nutrition and Self Care
- The impact of nutrition on physical and mental health
- Tips for developing a healthy relationship with food
- The importance of self care and how to

incorporate it into your routine

Chapter 7: Building a Fitness Routine

- How to design a fitness routine that works for you
- Tips for staying consistent with your exercise routine
- The benefits of tracking your progress

Chapter 8: Overcoming Challenges

- Common challenges people face when trying to improve themselves
- Strategies for overcoming obstacles and staying on track
- The importance of self compassion and resilience

Chapter 9: The Role of Community

- The benefits of finding a community of like minded individuals
- How to build a support system for your self improvement journey
- Overview of different types of fitness communities and how to find one that works for you

Chapter 10: Putting It All Together

- Recap of key takeaways from the book
- Tips for incorporating what you've learned into your daily life
- Final thoughts on the importance of self improvement and the gym

In "Stronger, Faster, Better: Mastering Your Life Through Fitness and Self-Improvement" you'll discover how the gym can be a powerful tool for self improvement. You'll learn about the benefits of physical exercise, goal setting, mindset, nutrition, and self care. You'll also discover strategies for building a fitness routine, overcoming challenges, and finding a supportive community. By the end of the book, you'll have a comprehensive understanding of how the gym can help you achieve your self improvement goals and live your best life.

Chapter 1: Introduction

Self improvement is a lifelong journey that we all embark on to become the best versions of ourselves. It involves making positive changes in different areas of our lives, such as our health, relationships, career, and personal growth. The gym is a valuable tool that can help us achieve our self improvement goals, whether it's building a stronger body, improving our mental health, or boosting our confidence.

In this book, we will explore the many ways the gym can contribute to our self improvement journey. We'll dive into the science behind physical exercise, its impact on mental health, and the benefits of a healthy lifestyle. You'll learn about the power of goal setting, the importance of mindset, and strategies for overcoming obstacles.

But first, let's take a step back and define self improvement. Self improvement is the process of making positive changes in various areas of your life to become a better version of yourself. It's about identifying your strengths and weaknesses and working towards enhancing your strengths while improving on your weaknesses. Self Improvement can take many forms, including physical, mental, emotional, spiritual, and social.

The benefits of self improvement are numerous. They include increased confidence, a sense of purpose, improved relationships, enhanced mental and physical health, and a greater sense of fulfilment. Self improvement is an ongoing process, and the journey itself is just as important as the destination.

The gym is a great place to start your self improvement journey. Physical exercise has been shown to improve mood, reduce stress, and increase cognitive function. Regular exercise can help you build a stronger body, improve your endurance, and increase your overall fitness level. The gym provides a supportive environment where you can challenge yourself and push yourself to new limits.

Throughout this book, we'll explore how the gym can help you achieve your self improvement goals, and we'll provide you with practical tips and advice for incorporating fitness into your daily routine. Whether you're a seasoned gym goer or a beginner, this book will provide you with the tools and knowledge you need to achieve your self improvement goals and become stronger every day.

Chapter 2: Understanding Self Improvement

Self improvement is a complex and multifaceted concept that encompasses many different areas of life. In this chapter, we'll explore what selfimprovement means, the benefits of self improvement, and the different areas of life that you can focus on to improve yourself.

Self Improvement can be defined as the process of making positive changes in various areas of your life to become a better version of yourself. It's a continuous journey that requires effort, dedication, and a willingness to grow and learn. Self Improvement is not about perfection or comparison to others, but rather about improving yourself in a way that is meaningful and fulfilling to you.

The benefits of self improvement are numerous. They include increased confidence, a sense of purpose, improved relationships, enhanced mental and physical health, and a greater sense of fulfilment. When you work on improving yourself, you become more resilient, adaptable, and better equipped to handle the challenges that life throws your way.

There are many different areas of life that you can focus on to improve yourself. These include:

- Physical Health: Taking care of your body through exercise, healthy eating, and self care is essential for overall well being. Improving your physical health can lead to increased energy, improved mood, and a stronger immune system.

- Mental Health: Mental health is just as important as

physical health. Improving your mental health can involve practices such as mindfulness, meditation, and therapy. By prioritising your mental health, you can reduce stress, anxiety, and depression.

- Personal Growth: Personal growth involves developing your skills, talents, and interests. This can include learning new skills, pursuing hobbies, or setting new challenges for yourself. By investing in personal growth, you can increase your self awareness and become more fulfilled.

- Relationships: Building strong and healthy relationships is a vital aspect of self improvement. By focusing on communication, trust, and empathy, you can enhance your relationships with family, friends, and colleagues.

- Career: Improving your career can involve setting new goals, pursuing further education or training, or seeking new opportunities. By advancing your career, you can increase your income, develop new skills, and find greater fulfilment in your work.

In this chapter, we've explored the meaning and benefits of self improvement and the different areas of life that you can focus on to improve yourself. By understanding what selfimprovement means and what it involves, you can begin to develop a plan for achieving your goals and becoming the best version of yourself.

Chapter 3: The Science of Exercise

The gym is a powerful tool for self improvement, and understanding the science behind physical exercise can help you maximise its benefits. In this chapter, we'll explore the many ways that exercise impacts the body and brain and why it's an essential component of self improvement.

Exercise is a form of physical activity that involves moving the body and increasing energy expenditure. It's a vital part of a healthy lifestyle and is essential for maintaining physical and mental health. Exercise can take many forms, including cardiovascular exercise, strength training, and flexibility training.

When you exercise, your body undergoes many changes at the cellular level. Exercise increases blood flow to the muscles, providing them with oxygen and nutrients to fuel movement. As a result, exercise helps to build stronger muscles, increase endurance, and improve overall physical fitness.

Exercise also has many benefits for mental health. Regular exercise has been shown to reduce stress and anxiety, improve mood, and boost cognitive function. Exercise triggers the release of endorphins, which are natural mood boosting chemicals that can reduce pain and increase feelings of happiness.

Beyond the physical and mental benefits, exercise has many other health benefits. It can improve cardiovascular health, reduce the risk of chronic diseases such as diabetes and heart disease, and increase longevity. Exercise can also improve sleep quality and help with weight management.

The benefits of exercise are numerous, but it's important to note that the type and intensity of exercise you engage in can impact the benefits you receive. High Intensity exercise has been shown to have greater benefits for cardiovascular health and weight management, while low intensity exercise can be beneficial for stress reduction and mental health.

Incorporating exercise into your daily routine can be challenging, but there are many strategies that can help you stay motivated and on track. Setting goals, finding an accountability partner, and making exercise a habit can all help you maintain a regular exercise routine.

In this chapter, we've explored the science of exercise and its many benefits for physical and mental health. By understanding the impact of exercise on the body and brain, you can begin to develop a fitness routine that maximises its benefits and supports your self improvement journey.

Chapter 4: The Gym and Self Improvement

The gym is a popular destination for those seeking to improve themselves physically, but it can also have a profound impact on other areas of life. In this chapter, we'll explore how the gym can support self improvement in various ways and provide tips for maximising its benefits.

Physical Health: The most obvious benefit of the gym is its impact on physical health. Regular exercise can help to build muscle, increase endurance, and improve cardiovascular health. By committing to a consistent gym routine, you can make meaningful improvements in your physical health that can support your overall wellbeing.

Mental Health: The benefits of the gym extend beyond physical health and can have a significant impact on mental health. Exercise has been shown to reduce stress and anxiety, improve mood, and boost cognitive function. By making the gym a regular part of your routine, you can support your mental health and wellbeing.

SelfConfidence: Improving your physical fitness can have a profound impact on self confidence. As you make progress in the gym, you'll start to see improvements in your physical appearance and feel more confident in your abilities. This increased confidence can translate into other areas of life, such as personal relationships and career.

GoalSetting: The gym is a great place to practise goal setting and develop discipline. By setting achievable goals, you can work towards something tangible and measure your progress. This process can help to build discipline and improve self motivation, both of which are essential for self improvement.

Community: The gym can also provide a sense of community and support. By attending regular gym classes or working with a personal trainer, you can connect with like minded individuals who share similar goals. This sense of community can be motivating and inspiring, providing an additional source of support for self improvement.

To maximise the benefits of the gym for self improvement, it's important to approach your workouts with intention and purpose. Set specific goals, vary your workouts to challenge yourself, and stay committed to your routine. Consider working with a personal trainer or attending group fitness classes to increase accountability and support.

In this chapter, we've explored the many ways that the gym can support self improvement, including its impact on physical and mental health, self confidence, goal setting, and community. By approaching the gym with intention and commitment, you can harness its power to support your self improvement journey.

Chapter 5: Overcoming Gym Anxiety

For many people, the thought of going to the gym can be overwhelming and intimidating. This feeling of anxiety can prevent individuals from starting or maintaining a gym routine, despite the numerous benefits. In this chapter, we'll explore strategies for overcoming gym anxiety and building confidence in the gym.

Understand Your Fear: The first step in overcoming gym anxiety is to identify the root cause of your fear. Common fears include feeling judged, feeling inexperienced or out of shape, or not knowing how to use the equipment. By understanding the specific cause of your anxiety, you can develop a plan to address it.

Start Small: If the thought of going to the gym is overwhelming, start with small steps. Consider going for a short walk or doing a home workout to build your confidence and familiarity with exercise. As you become more comfortable, gradually increase the intensity and duration of your workouts.

Educate Yourself: Learning about exercise and proper technique can help to build confidence and reduce anxiety. Consider working with a personal trainer or attending an orientation session at the gym to learn how to use the equipment properly and develop a safe and effective workout routine.

Find a Gym Buddy: Having a workout partner can provide accountability, support, and motivation. Consider finding a friend or family member who shares your fitness goals and attend the gym together.

Change Your Perspective: Rather than viewing the gym as a place of judgement or competition, reframe your perspective. The gym can be a place of self improvement and personal growth. By focusing on your own progress and goals, you can cultivate a sense of accomplishment and confidence.

Practise SelfCare: Prioritising selfcare, such as getting enough sleep, eating a healthy diet, and managing stress, can help to reduce anxiety and improve your overall well being. By taking care of your physical and mental health, you can build the resilience and confidence needed to overcome gym anxiety.

In this chapter, we've explored strategies for overcoming gym anxiety and building confidence in the gym. By understanding the root cause of your fear, starting small, educating yourself, finding a gym buddy, changing your perspective, and practising selfcare, you can build the confidence needed to harness the many benefits of the gym for self improvement.

Chapter 6: Incorporating the Gym into a Busy Lifestyle

One of the biggest challenges of going to the gym can be finding the time to fit it into a busy schedule. With work, family, and other obligations, it can be difficult to prioritise exercise. In this chapter, we'll explore strategies for incorporating the gym into a busy lifestyle and making exercise a consistent part of your routine.

Set Realistic Goals: When incorporating the gym into a busy lifestyle, it's important to set realistic goals. Consider your schedule and determine how much time you realistically have to commit to exercise. Set achievable goals that fit into your schedule and build gradually as you become more comfortable.

Schedule Your Workouts: Just as you would schedule an important meeting or appointment, prioritise your workouts by scheduling them into your calendar. By setting aside dedicated time for exercise, you can ensure that it becomes a consistent part of your routine.

MultiTask: Incorporate exercise into other parts of your day by finding ways to multitask. For example, consider biking or walking to work or running errands on foot. This can help to build physical activity into your daily routine and maximise your time.

Wake Up Earlier: While it can be difficult to wake up earlier, doing so can provide dedicated time for exercise before the rest of the day's obligations begin. Consider waking up an hour earlier to fit in a workout, or splitting your workout into two shorter sessions during the day.

Use Your Lunch Break: If you have a lunch break during the day, use it to fit in a quick workout. Consider going for a walk or doing a quick weightlifting session during your break.

Find a Gym Close to Work or Home: Finding a gym that is conveniently located can help to reduce the amount of time spent commuting and make it easier to fit exercise into a busy schedule.

In this chapter, we've explored strategies for incorporating the gym into a busy lifestyle, including setting realistic goals, scheduling workouts, multitasking, waking up earlier, using lunch breaks, and finding a conveniently located gym. By prioritising exercise and making it a consistent part of your routine, you can build physical and mental wellbeing and support self improvement, even in the midst of a busy lifestyle.

Chapter 7: The Importance of Rest and Recovery

When it comes to self improvement through exercise, it's important to remember that rest and recovery are just as important as the workout itself. In this chapter, we'll explore the importance of rest and recovery and strategies for incorporating them into your workout routine.

Why Rest and Recovery are Important: Rest and recovery allow your body time to repair and rebuild after exercise, and are essential for optimising physical and mental wellbeing. Without adequate rest and recovery, you may experience fatigue, burnout, and even injury.

Understanding the Types of Rest and Recovery: There are two types of rest and recovery: active and passive. Active recovery includes low intensity exercise, such as yoga or walking, that promotes blood flow and reduces muscle soreness. Passive recovery includes methods such as massage, foam rolling, and stretching, which can help to reduce muscle tension and promote relaxation.

Building Rest and Recovery into Your Routine: To incorporate rest and recovery into your workout routine, consider scheduling regular rest days, alternating between high intensity and low intensity workouts, and incorporating active and passive recovery methods. It's also important to prioritise sleep, nutrition, and stress management to support physical and mental wellbeing.

The Role of Mindfulness in Rest and Recovery: Mindfulness practices, such as meditation and deep breathing, can help to reduce stress and promote relaxation, which are essential for effective rest and recovery. Consider incorporating mindfulness practices into your rest and recovery routine to support mental wellbeing.

Monitoring Your Progress: Paying attention to your body and monitoring your progress can help to identify when rest and recovery are needed. If you are experiencing persistent fatigue, soreness, or other symptoms, consider taking a break from exercise or incorporating additional rest and recovery methods.

In this chapter, we've explored the importance of rest and recovery for self improvement through exercise. By understanding the types of rest and recovery, building them into your routine, prioritising sleep and stress management, incorporating mindfulness practices, and monitoring your progress, you can support physical and mental wellbeing and optimise the benefits of exercise.

Chapter 8: Overcoming Plateaus and Staying Motivated

One of the challenges of self improvement through exercise is overcoming plateaus and staying motivated over the long term. In this chapter, we'll explore strategies for breaking through plateaus and staying motivated to achieve your fitness goals.

Recognizing Plateaus: Plateaus occur when progress in your fitness goals slows or comes to a halt. This can be frustrating and demotivating, but it's important to remember that they are a normal part of the process.

Changing Up Your Routine: To overcome plateaus, consider changing up your workout routine. This can include trying new exercises, increasing intensity or duration, or incorporating strength training or high intensity interval training (HIIT) into your routine. By challenging your body in new ways, you can break through plateaus and continue making progress.

Setting New Goals: Setting new goals can help to provide motivation and a sense of purpose. Consider setting shortterm and longterm goals, such as running a 5K or completing a certain number of pushups, and tracking your progress to stay motivated.

Finding a Workout Partner: Working out with a partner can provide accountability and motivation, and can make workouts more enjoyable. Consider finding a friend, family member, or personal trainer to work out with.

Rewarding Yourself: Celebrate your progress and accomplishments by rewarding yourself with something that you enjoy, such as a massage or a favourite meal. This can help to reinforce positive behaviour and provide motivation to continue.

Finding Inspiration: Finding inspiration in the success of others, such as athletes or fitness influencers, can provide motivation and help to stay focused on your goals. Consider following fitness influencers on social media or joining a fitness community to connect with others who share similar goals.

In this chapter, we've explored strategies for overcoming plateaus and staying motivated to achieve your fitness goals, including changing up your routine, setting new goals, finding a workout partner, rewarding yourself, and finding inspiration. By staying motivated and persisting through plateaus, you can achieve your fitness goals and support overall physical and mental wellbeing.

Chapter 9: Building a Sustainable Fitness Routine

Creating a sustainable fitness routine is essential for long term success and overall well being. In this chapter, we'll explore strategies for building a fitness routine that is sustainable and enjoyable.

Assessing Your Current Routine: Before making any changes to your fitness routine, it's important to assess your current habits and identify areas for improvement. Consider tracking your workouts and assessing your progress, as well as identifying any obstacles that may be preventing you from staying consistent.

Setting Realistic Goals: Setting realistic goals that align with your lifestyle and fitness level is essential for building a sustainable routine. Consider setting both shortterm and longterm goals, and be sure to celebrate your progress along the way.

Finding Activities You Enjoy: Incorporating activities that you enjoy into your fitness routine can make it more sustainable and enjoyable. Consider trying a variety of activities, such as swimming, hiking, or dance classes, to find what you enjoy most.

Prioritising Recovery: Prioritising rest and recovery is essential for building a sustainable fitness routine. Incorporate rest days, active recovery, and passive recovery methods such as stretching and massage into your routine to support overall wellbeing.

Staying Accountable: Staying accountable to your fitness goals can help to ensure consistency and progress. Consider working with a personal trainer or joining a fitness community to provide accountability and motivation.

Making it a Lifestyle: Building a sustainable fitness routine requires making exercise a part of your lifestyle. Consider finding ways to incorporate movement into your daily routine, such as walking or biking to work, taking the stairs instead of the elevator, or incorporating stretching or yoga into your morning routine.

In this chapter, we've explored strategies for building a sustainable fitness routine, including assessing your current routine, setting realistic goals, finding activities you enjoy, prioritising recovery, staying accountable, and making exercise a part of your lifestyle. By building a sustainable fitness routine, you can achieve your fitness goals, support overall wellbeing, and enjoy the benefits of exercise for years to come.

Chapter 10: Overcoming Obtacles and Staying Consistent

Staying consistent with your fitness routine can be challenging, especially when obstacles arise. In this chapter, we'll explore strategies for overcoming obstacles and staying consistent with your fitness routine.

Identifying Obstacles: Identifying obstacles that may be preventing you from staying consistent with your fitness routine is the first step to overcoming them. Common obstacles may include lack of time, lack of motivation, or injury.

Planning Ahead: Planning ahead can help to overcome obstacles and ensure consistency with your fitness routine. Consider scheduling workouts in advance, preparing healthy meals and snacks ahead of time, and packing a gym bag the night before.

Adapting to Changes: Adapting to changes in your routine, such as travel or busy work periods, can be challenging but is essential for maintaining consistency. Consider finding ways to incorporate movement into your routine, such as doing bodyweight exercises in your hotel room or taking a walk during your lunch break.

Seeking Support: Seeking support from friends, family, or a personal trainer can provide motivation and accountability to help you stay consistent with your fitness routine. Consider finding a workout partner or joining a fitness community to connect with others who share similar goals.

Overcoming Mental Blocks: Overcoming mental blocks, such as negative self talk or fear of failure, is essential for staying consistent with your fitness routine. Consider practising positive self talk and setting realistic goals to help build confidence and motivation.

Celebrating Progress: Celebrating progress along the way can provide motivation and reinforce positive behaviour. Consider tracking your progress and celebrating milestones with rewards or by treating yourself to something you enjoy.

In this chapter, we've explored strategies for overcoming obstacles and staying consistent with your fitness routine, including identifying obstacles, planning ahead, adapting to changes, seeking support, overcoming mental blocks, and celebrating progress. By staying consistent and persisting through obstacles, you can achieve your fitness goals and support overall physical and mental wellbeing.

Synopsis

"Stronger, Faster, Better: Mastering Your Life Through Fitness and Self-Improvement" is a comprehensive guide to help individuals improve their physical and mental wellbeing through fitness. The book is divided into ten chapters, covering a range of topics from the benefits of exercise and nutrition to building a sustainable fitness routine and overcoming obstacles.

In the first chapter, readers are introduced to the benefits of fitness and how it can improve their overall quality of life. Chapter two explores the importance of setting goals and creating a plan to achieve them. In chapter three, readers learn about the role of nutrition in achieving their fitness goals, including the importance of a balanced diet and hydration.

Chapter four covers the different types of exercises, including cardio, strength, and flexibility, and how to incorporate them into a fitness routine. Chapter five provides tips for staying motivated and developing a positive mindset. In chapter six, readers learn about the benefits of working with a personal trainer or joining a fitness community for additional support and accountability.

Chapter seven explores the importance of rest and recovery, including the benefits of stretching, massage, and sleep. In chapter eight, readers learn about the importance of tracking progress and measuring success. Chapter nine provides strategies for building a sustainable fitness routine, including finding activities that you enjoy, prioritising recovery, and making exercise a part of your lifestyle.

Finally, chapter ten covers how to overcome obstacles and stay consistent with your fitness routine, including planning ahead, seeking support, and celebrating progress.

Overall, "Stronger, Faster, Better: Mastering Your Life Through Fitness and Self-Improvement" provides a comprehensive and practical guide for individuals looking to improve their physical and mental wellbeing through fitness. With the knowledge and strategies provided in this book, readers can create a sustainable fitness routine that supports their overall health and wellbeing.